ISBN 13-9781467978477
Cover Design: Naiser Design Agency
Printing in the United States of America
First Printing Date: 10-05-05
Second Printing Date: 11-15-08
Copyright 2008 by Greg Ryan

website: www.resolutions.bz
Blogs: www.resolutionsblog.com
www.gregryanfitness.com

About the Author

At age 45, Greg Ryan's career began thirty years ago as a professional fitness trainer. In 1986 he won his first of two Michigan bodybuilding championships. He won his second title in 1988. In 1990 he moved to Los Angeles California, where his knowledge enthusiasm and skill attracted the attention of fitness guru Kathy Smith.

During this time Greg ran one of the largest personal training businesses in LA. Attracting numerous high profile movies stars such as Brooke Shields, Bridget Fonda, Connie Sellecca and many more. Greg built a reputation for exercise and behavior change and in the fall of 1992 appeared on the Today Show and Good Morning America.

In 1994 Greg returned to college to further his knowledge in Physical Therapy. During this time Greg's gift of motivating individuals led him to production of his own television segment on FOX TV. 1997 Greg relocated to Louisville Kentucky were he built and operated a private clinic specializing in obesity and diabetic weight loss programs.

Numerous bodybuilding titles, movie star clients, over a dozen authored books and counting; this has made him one of the most experienced and sought after experts in the business. Today Greg has acquired almost a hundred thousand hours of personal training to go with his well rounded career.

Why should you read this book?

From the Author

As a health club owner I made most of my money between Jan 1 and April 30. Why? Because people like you set New Years Resolutions and broke them time and time again.

I'm writing this book to teach you why you break them and how to achieve them; quit throwing your money away at health clubs, stop failing at your fitness goals for ever. Read on…

Content

Introduction

Four questions we will answer:

Why do you set New Years Resolutions in the first place?

Why do you break them?

How do you set a New Years Resolution guaranteed not to fail?

How do you set a fool proof plan to achieve them?

New Year's Resolutions are only as good as the willingness you have in changing your present habits. You have to be willing to pay a small price in hope that you do not pay a much larger one later. So I ask, **"What price are you willing to pay for good health and a better quality of life?"**

Most say, *"I will do whatever it takes to be healthy,"* yet months later, off the wagon you go. What's it going to take for you to stick to your goals?
Most important when are you going to address the question,

Why Am I Waiting?

I know it and you know it, deep down the heart needs to change before anything else will. And I truly think you know that the reason for your current health status has to do more with **laziness, denial** and **pride** than anything.

No one will make the decision to exercise and eat better for you, nor can anyone believe in you enough to make this happen; you alone have that already inside you. In order to find that first, have to be willing to accept the situation "as it is" and then ask for assistance with it. This coming year can be different if you chose to make it different.

Thirty days! The doctor says there's not anything else they can do, what the heck does that mean, their doctors for God sakes? "Jesus, I have a maybe a month to live Greg, what do I do now?" What don't you do, Benny? I whispered.

For the next three hours he laid there in that hospital bed speaking of every reason why he didn't quit, every excuse he ever made and now all he could do, all he had the strength to do was fight back the tears from fear and guilt he had harbored for so long.

Where were those feelings just a few hours ago, last month or last year, I thought? Even though we all had our own crosses to bear we still spoke often that the cigs may kill someday if he didn't stop.

Yet, what could I do, I filled my own life up with worry, resentment, pride and guilt; all different types of cancer.

Did I have the right to ask him to quit when I, in a different way wasn't willing to quit listening to my own demons that were eating at me on the inside.

Why did Benny wait until it was too late too quit smoking? Why does it take a threatening event in order to wake us up? What do you say to those whose life's has just been cut short; the only thing I could do was reflect?

Benny all I can say is, *live life while you have it the best way you know how,* but all the while I new I was not speaking so much to him as I was to me. What would I to do, what could I do? Why wait to tell someone I love or forgive them? Why wait to make a difference in my family's life or others? Why wait to do something about my health?

If I needed a push I got it, I saw it right there in that bed, in the eyes and in the heart of a man that was only going to have moments to live.

1
The Push
(Why we set them)

Q: Why do I set a New Years Resolution?

A: For the smell of it- Because You Can!

A part of the enjoyment of getting a new car lies on the inside. More often you wash it a lot, worry about dings on the outside, but one of the best things in getting a new car is the new car smell on the inside. You get in, take a deep breathe and it's fresh and clean. In some way you feel a sense of accomplishment and welcoming change in your life yet, it all seems to disappear soon after, why?

Could it be we set New Year's Resolutions for the *smell* of it? You need a new start, something to take care of, nurture and call it your own. So out of the blue you half heartedly set a goal for the year regarding your health. Maybe you do it for other reasons like...

A: For the *Symbolism* of it- It's Trendy!

Being hip and trendy seems to be the thing these days, people want to fit in and be apart of something; pressure surrounds you no matter age, economic level or Geographic's. Being cool use to be what kind of car you had or what style hand bag you carried, today anything can be considered cool. *Could setting a New Years resolution be considered hip?* Silly yes, but I do think some people set them just to fit in?

Think about it, what does it feel like when you do something just because someone else is doing it; not very fore filling is it; maybe even depressing?

A: For Post Partum Blues- Avoid Depression!

The holidays bring family dysfunction, emotions and even weight gain. Once all the excitement has left, what's usually there, leftover food, excess weight and a sense of let down?
You need something to pick you up so maybe you set a New Years Resolution because you are depressed.

The average person gains five to seven pounds between Thanksgiving and New Years.

That same person keeps it on like interest payments on the credit card, never paying it off, later buyers' remorse sets in and you feel let down, so what do you do? You figure the best way to get out of the funk is to start over; these are all good intentions! However, twelve months later it's déjà vu same feelings, same problem.

<u>Rule #1</u>
Don't set a New Years Resolution!

Have you ever said,

"Well I'll put off doing the laundry until tomorrow," or *"I'll pay off the credit card next month?"*

What happens, you usually don't end up doing what you said?

Even though we set resolutions the key is to get to a point when you don't need to set one. What do I mean? When you put off starting something that says you're really not serious or don't have a grasp of the importance of situation. You may be able to get by with not paying the bill or the pile of laundry, but putting off a heart attack or stroke or diabetes is out of your control and unpredictable. I hope someday you don't have to set a New Years Resolutions because you have been taking care of yourself all year long.

For most, the New Years Resolutions is just a part of the year that gives you hope. It doesn't matter what the reasons are for setting them, it's more important to determine *why* you continually fall off the wagon. For some reason each year you have great intentions, yet the motivation goes away. Let's look the why's.

2
The Problem!
(Why we break them)

Q: Why do I break resolutions?

There is always a reason for not following through on things we start. If I were a psychologist I would tell you it's probably one or all of three things; *fear, resentment and or denial.*

A: Fear- Illusions in the head

For some, it may be a fear of failure or even accomplishment. In the past you failed to follow through so you have convinced yourself this time would be no different. Opposite of that would be the fear of success. *What if I succeed and reached my goal, how could I maintain that, how could I measure up?* Just think about that, how stupid does that sound? Fear is a big manipulator.

<u>Fear</u>- **F**alse **E**vidence **A**ppearing **R**eal.

Resentment

Could you be mad because of the very fact you have to set a Resolution to get motivated? You resent having to work on your health; you wish you were back in the same shape at twenty?

A: Denial

Are you flat out denying your health? You admit you're a few pounds over weight, but can't come to grips with really how seriously out of shape you are. We can justify anything. Denial is really dangerous.

A: Easy Outs- Are you serious enough?

Let's say you're having dinner with a friend and this is the last time you will ever see them again, what do you say? Would you speak of superficial things, would you be in a hurry? I'm sure you would try to cherish every moment and talk about more meaningful things, wouldn't you? Time, relationships and material things are all parts of life we take for granted.

Have you even taken a New Year's Resolution for granted? Have you ever thought that there will be another one next year so why try this time?

A: Scarty Cat!

Have you ever noticed how cats behave when you want them around, they avoid you like the plague? But, when you aren't noticing they're right under your nose.

When setting resolutions you have to be careful not to set yourself up for failure; this happens when your expectations are higher than the responsibilities you have in your life.

If you notice there's an attitude shift from December 31st to January 1st, people think they can easily go from not exercising at all to working out five days a week. While noble as that may sound, the brain is laughing; based on your past performance the brain can not conceive going from nothing to regular exercise. So it just laughs and thinks, "*Are you nuts?*"

When this happens you sabotage your goals and run from them like a scared cat. Do the work and the rest will follow!

A: Don't sleep on it- Where's your sense of urgency?

One day while having lunch I met a guy who was in his early forties, he quit smoking two packs a day after twenty years, just like that.

"How did you do it, if you don't mind me asking? Did you just wake up one morning and say that's it?"

He said, "I didn't have to wake up. It was ten years ago next month. I met a gentlemen who suffered from infasemia. And said, that's it, I will never smoke another cigarette again. And I have not had one or the urge since." It was just like that? I asked. Just like that, he said.

Achieving your New Years Resolutions is more of a mind set than a numbers game.

A: Breaking the Barriers

Most everyone has a fear of something and at times can think too much by analyzing it to death; the bottom line is barriers keep us from starting and finishing Resolutions. The truth is they are just illusions, they're not real. If you figure out what you're afraid of, resentful toward or in denial of, chances are you can break through them.

For most getting started is not the tallest hurdle, staying the course is. Motivation is much easier at the beginning, but the river of new found energy runs dry a few months later. Let's look at ways to increase our staying power, our ability to stay focused on the intentions that start off so great. It really does start with a good sound decision from the heart.

When a meaningful decision is made it's almost impossible to turn back. Sure you make excuses, but your heart doesn't buy into them, so you keep going.

Rule 2
Don't give yourself an easy way out!

You have to put some sort of seriousness to your desires or you will eventually find ways to get out of the commitment. There has to be consequences to your in actions.

3
The Prep Work
(How to set a Resolution)

Q: How do I set them?

A: Mind Set- Goals change decisions don't!

If this coming year is going to be any different you are going to have to think differently. I have a motto that says, *"There are no more options!"* What do I mean by this? You have to come too a point in your life where all the excuses and are not good anymore and you have no choice, but to move ahead. Sure you do have a choice however the consequences are so severe that you can not afford to take that chance any longer.

One day I came to that place where I had no more options left; I decided that if I did not change my thinking, behavior and habits, it would someday cost me my life. My family was full of diabetes, strokes, depression and just plain bad attitudes.

Did I want that for myself? No. So I had one choice, and that was to move ahead one day at a time.

Looking back twenty five years ago the last thing in the world I thought was becoming an author, bodybuilder, business owner or at the very least a consistent exerciser. What I did know was that if I kept going something had to happen to my body and to my mind. The exercising just had to pay off.

A: Goal Setting- Keep them realistic!

Set one major goal for the year that you ultimately strive for. Most people go out too fast, look around and don't know what direction they are headed in. It is vital that you not just set a goal, but always keep the big picture in mind.

A: Big Picture Goals

Three elements of attaining long term goals; hope, belief and *pure* motives.

Hope

"You can live a month without food. You can live a week without water, you can live five minutes without air, but you cannot live a second without HOPE." If you have just a small bit of hope it can keep you going for a day. I always believed that no one has a

right to take your hope away, whether you choose to let them may be another story.

Belief

Life was scary for me growing up. I was afraid of not meeting the expectations of those around me. I didn't know what direction to take in life or what advice to follow. When I first stepped into a health club, it was equally as frightening. I had two friends that exercised with me on a regular basis.

The confidence they had in me started positively affecting my attitude and fear of failure. After awhile, I noticed those fears slowly began disappearing.

With a little bit of hope, mixed with some faith, I knew I could really make things happen. Everyone can have hope but it's much harder to have belief in yourself, especially when you are unsure of the outcome; not sure if you're going to succeed or fail.

This is a process, but what I have noticed is each day builds on its own. Now I look back and think, well if I did that I surely can do this. I already proved too myself I could accomplish something. Action builds belief in one self.

As I developed more confidence, I started to realize how important it was for change to come from the inside out. Looking better, having more energy and getting physically stronger are great, but what I am most grateful for is that of my heart. I felt better about myself. That heart-felt motivation becomes the glue that has kept you going for years.

No matter what goals you set keep this in mind; you have got to be in this for the long haul. Deep inside you need to do this for the right reasons if not, sooner or later you will lose motivation and stop.

Now, you must understand there will never be a perfect synario for you. In order to get through the little things you have to keep the big picture in mind. What does the big picture look like for you? Does it look like a perfect body or does it look like a better quality of life?

A: Seasonal Goals

When you have a main goal established now work backwards with seasonal ones. These are small incremental goals, usually in three month segments. Be sure to make them progressive in nature, building up to your main year end goal.

A: Weekly Goals

Some people have a hard time even thinking in three month segments, if so, set weekly goals. Do what ever it takes to get there.

In the beginning like I said, I couldn't even think that far ahead, just let me accomplish my daily one first.

A: Realistic Goals

A major mistake is to set an unrealistic goal based on your lifestyle and present situation. I can not over estimate this enough. In some situations your responsibilities may not allow you to set lofty goals. You may have to take a step back and set smaller ones in order to attain them at that particular point in your life.

It is smarter to set realistic goals, attain them and get to your destination eventually rather than to try to shoot for the moon, missing.

A: Keep the ball rolling- All momentum!

This one never crosses people's minds until it's too late. In order not to lose momentum pre-plan your goals. You have already somewhat done so by setting seasonal goals.

However what happens is a let down between goals may occur, once you have achieved one.

As you come up on attaining a goal, start thinking and strategizing how you are going to attain the next seasonal goal. But, keep in mind not to lose sight of your present one; that is your main focus.

My point is to keep the momentum moving by staying ahead of the game, by planning your path ahead of time. It's sure a lot easier steering a car while it's moving rather than turning the wheel while it sits it in a parking.

A: The Power behind the Pen- Write them down!

I can not totally explain why writing your goal's down is such a powerful exercise, but it is. I have experienced it first hand that when you write down your goals over and over again, transformations take place first in your mind and then within your body.

When I became a champion bodybuilder, four months prior to the day of my competitions I wrote down on a piece of paper, *"I am Mr. Michigan 1988"* at least one hundred times. I can not to this day explain how it happened but over time the pen convinced my body to achieve that goal. It is impossible to build a solid house on sand, it needs a foundation.

Writing your goals down can seem painful at times, however, later on it you get a sense of direction, and a deep feeling that you're on the right path. With this comes a much greater need and want to see it through. Writing goals down will not make the path any easier, but it very possibly will make it straighter.

<u>Rule 3</u>
The Goal may change, but your Decision will not!

Tip:
Set the Goal, decide and not look back

4
The Path
(How to achieve a Resolution)

Q: How do I achieve them?

A: Your Biggest Enemy- YOU!

The biggest enemy you have standing in the way of your success is not the French fries, ice cream or the scale- the biggest obstacle is your mind. If you are like most, you talk yourself out of everything. If you give yourself anytime to ponder you'll come up with the stupidest, most illogical reason NOT to get healthier and exercise.

The ones who have successfully kept weight off, lowered their body-fat levels, and dropped their blood pressure are the ones who did not wait for a perfect time. No perfect times, but there are big regrets.

A: You have to go from denial to having a desire.

What does it mean to have deep desire for something?

Remember those feelings you had back when you wanted your first bicycle. That Barbie doll you made a fit over in the toy store in front of everyone. Or what about that girl or boy you would have done just about anything for? There was such a hunger, a burning in your gut. You couldn't even think straight, eat or sleep because it occupied your every thought. You just had to have it!

A: Desperado

One day I was having lunch with a buddy when through the front door she walked. I took a deep breath, leaned over to my friend and said, "I have never done this before; it's not my style; it's totally out of my comfort zone and for the life of me I do not understand why I am doing it, I JUST HAVE TO, even if I make a fool out of myself.

I stood up, grabbed the closest waitress (not literally) and said, *"I have to meet that woman that just sat down over there. Buy her lunch and tell her it is a random act of kindness."*

Yeah, right. There was nothing random about it, I was on a mission. I was fueling a deep desire in my gut. I had never believed in love at first sight, until then.

Maybe I was at the "no options left" point in my life. Maybe I was being desperado, I don't know. I did not care. I just knew that I could not deny that physical, emotional burning, that hunger, that deep desire to know her. At that point, all fear, all logic and all common sense were covered up by the strong urge to move forward. But not all of you have a love story to tell, yet there are things in all of us that give you the potential of having that deep desire

A: Have Hope

Have hope! Accepting and acknowledging your health does not mean you have to give up hope, it can mean just the opposite,
"A new, fresh beginning." Many people have done extraordinary things with nothing but a little bit of hope; they arose every morning just hoping that that day would be better than the last.

A: Have an Open Mind

Have an open mind to exercise and better eating, rather than resenting it.

There aren't many people that get up and just can't wait to jump on a treadmill, and if you truly recent the fact that your health is bad you'll find it's harder to get started.

Accept that life will not hand you a perfect situation. If you think that the process will be smooth sailing or close to perfect, realize that's not going to happen.

Learn that your self-worth is not based upon if you ask for help along the way; we age, our metabolism slows down, and we are more prone to injuries.

A: Have a Long-Term Attitude

If you want to go from denial your health to having a desire you're going to go at it with an *all or nothing* attitude. If you are going to start now, you have to start for good. The reality is you will have good and bad attitude days, but understand, if you are going to be healthier through exercise and eating, you are going to have to participate in some form of exercise till the day you die. *This is not a temporary fix to a long-term problem; it is a lifestyle.*

A: Take an "Inside-Out" Approach

You will not win the aging battle if you think that all you have to do is work on the outside. When your motives and desires come from the heart or **"INSIDE-OUT"**, then true health begins to grow. And if your physical appearance changes during the process, that is icing on the cake. **Changing from the "INSIDE-OUT"** is a concept or idea, a day-to-day mindset.

Maybe that is why those that change for the good are those who decide right then and there to do so? They are the ones who ask themselves, "Why am I waiting?"

"Why are you waiting?"

Rule 4
Have a little Hope, Faith, and a Deep Desire!

5
The Prelude
(Why we wait)

Q: What happens if I wait?

If you knew today that during your next doctor's visit he would say,

"Too late! Nothing you can do now! Maybe if you would have started six months ago or a year. But, not now. There is nothing we can do for you unless you start getting some exercise."

Would you start to exercise? The truth is you're not promised tomorrow. I know that sounds like a cliché and I am no doctor, but what does that have anything to do with it? Nothing!

A: You get the "Lab Coat" Syndrome

It's really frustrating to see people take doctors more serious than *me* the fitness expert. We both share and suggest the same advice about exercise, but it's what the lab coat symbolizes that makes the difference; authority, sickness, even death makes you take it more serious.

I see people losing weight after they visit the doctor's office and I ask them, *"What did the doctor,"* and I scratch my head, thinking, *"Didn't I say the same thing to you for the last year?"* Maybe I should start wearing a lab coat.

A: You get the harsh facts.

If you are over forty, one out of three of you will break a bone, half of you will be obese and develop diabetes, and your children will be the first generation not to live to your age of death. This is sad but truth. Is this a scare tactic? Sure it is, if it gets you to start thinking and getting to move. Don't think for one second you're exempt from illness or an accident?

A: When there are no more options left

On any given day I have use every excuse not to exercise. I have come up with more reasons not to feel better than I can count. I don't know if there are any more options left for me to use. What happens when you run out of excuses? I have yet to hear someone give me a legitimate reason why NOT to exercise and eat better. And I doubt if you can come up with one yourself.

A: You Hit Rock Bottom

In my experience people throw the waiting game out the window when something of value is threatened to be taken from them. Why does it have to come to that in life though?

Why does it take something bad happening or losing someone you love in order to make you realize how serious your health is? Are you going to have to hit rock bottom in order to not wait any longer in starting?

You know it doesn't have to come to that, you can start today by asking yourself, *"What's next?"*

Rule 5
Don't think so much!

If you focus too much on the detail you will defeat yourself every time. We can come up with any reason NOT to do something.

6
The Present
(Taking the Next step)

Q: What's next?

What is next? Are you going to make fluffy, superficial pipe dream goals this year? Maybe it's the middle of summer and there are just too many other more important things to do, maybe its winter and just too cold. How about starting now? How about changing your life for ever? How about doing it the right way for once?

A: What was next for me?

I am forty- two years old, and growing up was a much different life than what it is today for me. I was a loner, overweight, low self esteem kid with no direction in my life. My exercise came from working on the farm sixteen hours a day.

Then one day, exercise and eating right found me; yes it found me. For you, I would suggest you find them before the hospital finds you. Make a long story short, the two of them, exercise and eating right, ended up changing that boy forever.

Could I have found in school what they gave me, no way? Could I have bought it on a midnight information commercial? Not on your life. Exercise and eating right not only gave me a stellar career, but it also saved my life. It gave me life. It changed me from the INSIDE OUT!

I'm not that insecure little kid anymore. I would say, I am in pretty descent shape too. And most importantly, they taught me that; this world and no one in it has the right to take my self esteem away from me.

It's not the bodybuilding champions, movie star clients or the best selling books that I carry with me everyday that matters most—what fills me up is what exercise and eating right has done for my heart and soul.

What keeps me going? I don't want to go back. Do I feel better, sure I do? Is my health better for exercising and eating right? Absolutely! But, what gets me up everyday realizing this is just a way of life – it's knowing I will never be the same again. I will never go back the person I once was.

I don't want to go back; I want so desperately to find out what I can be. And the only way of doing that is to get up and workout out again tomorrow.

What's next for you? Only you can answer that question. Where do you stand? Are you going back, or is this time different? Are you willing to make the sacrifices now in order to feel better in the future?

My challenge to you is to look forward with great anticipation, move forward with on wavering dedication, and to be willing to change while doing both.

A: Your next step

Changing ones weight and eating habits lies not in the products but in the minds. So I took what I had learned over the last two decades and put in on paper.

What I suggest is that your next step is to take this next section to heart. Here is my answer to America's health problem it is called;

CHANGING FROM THE
"INSIDE-OUT"

Through Real Behavior Change, Smarter Eating and Effective Exercising!

The secret to changing your weight and over all health's lies not so much in exercise charts, menus or health clubs, the answers are found in the......

Approach!

Rule 6
Changing the heart changes the waistline!

7
The Plan

Q: What is the right Approach?

The "**INSIDE-OUT**" approach to fitness differs from that of conventional wisdom. Most programs work on diet and exercise alone. They give suggestions on what foods to eat through recipes, calorie-counting books, and exercise tips. While this way may work in the short run, eventually your desire to get in better shape disappears.

In order to change your attitude and unwanted behaviours, there are three things you must learn:

- *How and what motivates you?*
- *What are the reasons behind your unwanted behaviors?*
- *What kind of support system is good for you?*

The "**INSIDE-OUT**" approach consists of five areas referred to as layers of learning:

Layer 1: _Awareness_ – *Be aware of your motives*

Layer 2: _Acceptance_ –*Swallow the facts*

Layer 3: _Assistance_ – *Ask for help*

Layer 4: _Appetite_ – *Balance and control*

Layer 5: _Activity_ – *Just Move it*

A: The Circle to Life

The **"INSIDE-OUT"** approach is an on-going process. In theory, it is a simple common sense idea. In practice, it will take hope, faith in your self and patience. To get the most out it, you may have to revisit some of the topics daily and at the very least, continue to keep the concept in mind all the time.

The goal is for you to develop a lifestyle that reflects this way of thinking.

There is no right or wrong way. Each slice of the pie builds on the others in a continuously and in many directions.

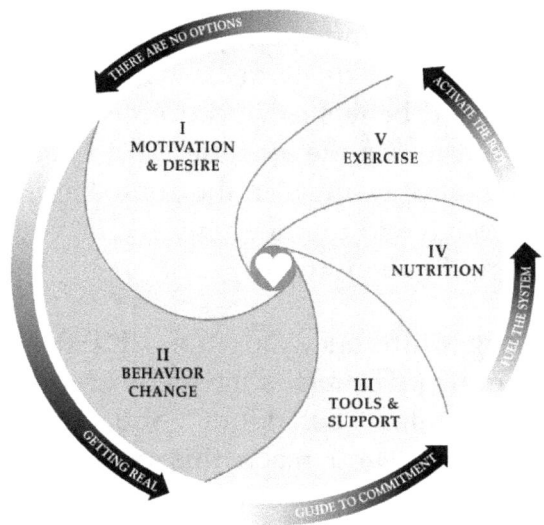

The *"Circle to Life"* is an illustration of how important each area is in relation to the other.

Being *aware* of your types of motives helps build and *accept* change in your behaviors. Getting *assistance* with your commitment feeds the *appetite* for good balanced food. Being more *active* promotes long-range success. Success breeds more motivation.

Keep in mind that all parts are necessary in order to make the most out of any health and fitness program.

A: Here is the difference.

The **"INSIDE-OUT"** concept takes a look at your exercise and eating behaviors through a *cognitive* approach. It deals with your motives, desires, and beliefs toward exercise and food. If you want to change attitudes and habits toward exercise and eating for the long haul, you are going to have to dig deep into WHY you feel the way you do about them.

The big difference in the "INSIDE- OUT" program from others is the focus on the motives, the unwanted behaviors, and the support system. Until you reach this point emotionally you will not take your health seriously long term.

You will continue to make New Years Resolutions only to feel like you are going nowhere with no purpose. So I ask, "What is your purpose with your health?"

8
The Purpose
(Expanding or Contracting)

Q: Are you Expanding or Contracting?

Chances are if you are forty years or over you are *contracting*, at least your life is as you know it. The world you live in is getting smaller. The body is not living up to the expectations and your mind tends to take the easier way out with the path of least resistance.

The problem with so called contracting is you are dying and don't even realize it. Your insides are emotionally rotting and either resentment, anger, or even depression eventually sets in. Then all you end up with is some form of regret.

Expansion- No Regrets

Why are you waiting? Do you want to be up in heaven someday looking back on your life and see all the things you regret NOT doing? I don't! But, you will if you continue to not get exercise or break a New Years Resolution. Get busy living or get busy dying! Contract or expand your life in other words.

Why Wait?
STEP #1
Don't set a New Years Resolution!

WHY DO I SET THEM?

Why do I want to set a New Years Resolution this year?

How do I feel when making New Years Resolutions?

What do I expect to get out of setting a New Years Resolutions?

Why do I feel this year will be different?

STEP #2
Don't give yourself an easy out!

GOALS change, DECISIONS do not!

Why Do I *Break* Them?

In the past I have broken my New Years Resolutions because:

What things can I do this year to prevent me from breaking the resolutions again?

Step #3
The Goal may change, but your Decision too will not!

How Do I *Set* Them?

If I had one and only one goal to make for the rest of my life concerning my health it would be?

This time next year what one goal am I going to have accomplished?

STEP #4
Have a little Hope, Faith, and a Deep Desire!

HOW DO I ACHIEVE THEM?

In a perfect world how do I want to feel and look like physically?

How long am I willing to work hard without expecting any results?

1 week

3 months

6 months

1 year

My motivation to exercise has more to do with my

- **looks**
- **internal vital signs?**

My hope for exercising is?

<u>Step #5</u>
Don't think so much, just do!

Why Wait?

What is the main reason for me not to start exercising and eating right today?

Do you believe your situation has to be perfect before you can start?

<u>Step #6</u>
Change from the Inside Out!

New Year's Commitment

I _____, by signing this commitment am promising myself that this year is going to be different.

I will continue to look at the big picture of good internal health, realistic goals and expectations.

I will ask for help if need be and have a one day at a time attitude. I also acknowledge that my health status is serious stuff. It is important to make it a top priority in my life no matter what. My health is my responsibility and no one else's.

Participant

Date

STEP #7
Determine your motives!

How are you motivated?

Are you fearful of your weight gain over the holidays?

By feeling better?

By looking better?

By an upcoming sporting event?

By an upcoming party event or vacation?

STEP #8
Discover the reasons for your unwanted behaviors!

The Iceberg Affect

The reason you break resolutions is because you don't deal with the deep issues that lie underneath. Like an iceberg, you only see a bit of your real reasons.

Above the surface:
What do you see?

Your unwanted behaviors

The unwanted behavior and the emotion that is usually attached to it are the two issues you encounter everyday.
Maybe it's not being able to start an exercising program or maybe it's not following through with one. Or, it could be eating too much at each meal.

Your emotions

An outward reaction to a behavior has an emotion attached to it. It could be a positive or a negative emotion, such as feeling guilty about eating too much and being physically uncomfortable.

One of my unwanted behaviors is;

Below the surface:
What don't you see?

Your Thoughts

Your emotions are attached to thoughts in your head.
Your thoughts can be broken down into two areas: what you SAY you believe and what the real TRUTH is!

What do you say you believe?

This area is where denial happens. You blame your unwanted behavior toward exercise on this or that to make yourself feel better.
Sometimes those beliefs can be just illusions, self-fabrications, and negative talk-- anything other than the facts. *Gosh, that food was good. I did not want that food to go to waste.* Statements like that are easy and partially true.

What do you say you believe about this unwanted behavior?

What is the real truth?

The real truth is what your core beliefs say about exercise. In most cases, it's fear. Fear of failure, success or looking dumb. "If I start to exercise, I may not follow through and I would consider it another failure in my life. If I do not clean my plate, I will get grounded as I did when I was a child." Thoughts like that come to mind, but the reality is none of those thoughts are true. You only think they are.

What is the real truth or reason behind your unwanted behavior!

STEP #9
Develop a GREAT support system!

Who are some trust worthy people you can put on your team?

What is a reward you can strive for?
Who is one person that can be my accountability partner?

Decide that food is not the problem!

Proper Planning Prevents Poor Performance!

The bottom line is food is not necessarily the root of the problem with your weight. It is the thought and lifestyle patterns behind them.

Here are the five P's check lists:

1. What is your Perspective on food?

- Eat to live.
- Live to eat.

Eat to live has a better outcome.

2. How often do you Pre-Plan your week of food?

- Never
- Sometimes
- All the time

Pre–planning weeks of food promotes better choice making.

3. Do you monitor your <u>Portions?</u>

- Never
- Sometimes
- All the time

Learning when to walk away from the table will save you many pounds a year.

4. Do you have food eating <u>patterns</u>?

- Never
- Sometimes
- All the time

Mixing food types up helps you're your metabolism going.

5. Do you find advertisements punch your buttons to eat when not even hungry?

- Never
- Sometimes
- All the time

Learning to recognize hot buttons saves money and pounds.

JUST *MOVE* IT!
<u>STEP #11</u>
Dedicate yourself to being active!

Lead, follow or get out of the way.

When setting resolutions I tend to:

- Be a perfectionist
- Set too high expectations
- Let pride keep me from starting

The key to following through this year is to keep your eye on the big picture. If you don't, the details will become a quicksand pit. The big picture is:

JUST MOVE IT!

The big picture is about being realistic with not too high of expectations and to focus on internal health issues, such as blood pressure, body fat, cholesterol levels, and a quiet mind.

STEP #12
Do not wait, start today!

Things to think about –Making it all work!

First: Take this seriously!

Second: Make a game plan, take one step at a time and follow through.

Third: Have some hope that it will work for you this time.

Forth: Get support from an honest, faithful friend.

Fifth: Decide that you are going to change your behaviors this time, no matter how hard it may become.

Sixth: Realize changing from the INSIDE OUT is the only long term way of reaching your New Years Resolutions!

Seventh: Realize and recognize sabotaging barriers keeping you from following through on your goals.

Conclusion

Ok! No more options, but to move forward. Flip a switch and look ahead not backwards. Last year, does not equal this year, and failure is only if you don't start.

Nothing wrong with goal setting, just do it realistically. Don't give yourself so many easy way outs and find some quality support around you. Success is not that hard, it just takes determination, belief and a day to day attitude. If can do it so you can.

Thank You

Thank you for reading, Why Wait. I wish you all the blessings in the world this coming year. I trust you have retained something of importance in making your health better.

As a token of my gratitude I have also included one of my e books on Lowering your Body-Fat! I hope you enjoy it, get something from it and apply it.

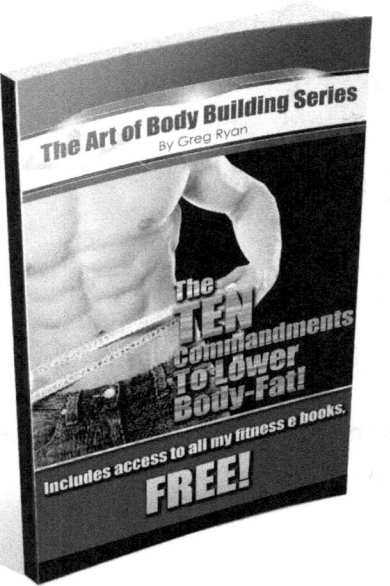

From the Author - My Story

I have kept my body-fat lower than fourteen percent for almost thirty years. This may not sound so remarkable to you, but to me it's been a life saver. You don't know it, but my family is full of diabetes, obesity, heart disease, depression and for one to beat those odds for so long, is not easy. However, this was not always so! It has been a struggle to say the least.

Fat Little Kids

I grew up with very little self-esteem or respect for my health. As a farm boy you have a built in activity regiment in daily farm chores, but that's as far as the exercise went. There's a difference between having to do something and wanting to. I just didn't want to do anything.

Fitness found me over time and so did a certain attitude that I would like to share in the next few pages. For what ever reason from day one in the gym I believed a persons body-fat levels were true indicators of fitness.

I also believed as a true body builder keeping your body-fat levels low as possible through the off seasons and year round was the ultimate. Any one can gain size, weight and even muscle, but not everyone can have the ideal balance of muscle to fat year after year; but I made a decision early on to try, and boy I'm glad I did.

Why you should read this e book!

This e book is not like most articles on health, fitness and even body-fat. This book is solely based off of my experience over the last thirty years and what worked for me.

Any guy can put on muscle size and any woman can get thin, but few can get their body-fat levels low and maintain it.

Contents

Introduction

Too many people focus on the scale, and in the end lose the battle mentally and physically. If you pants are lose, muscles defined and tight, why do you care what the scale registers? Any body can lose or gain weight, but a much less percentage of people keep their body-fat at a respectable level. And very few can maintain it lower than normal for years, I did.

No matter what your age, keeping a lower level of body-fat is vital. If you are of the younger generation then you look better if you are a baby boomer or older a lower fat level is an extremely healthier state of being. This e book outlines just a few ways I have kept my body-fat low for many years. Don't be fooled by the length or lack of gimmicky phrases, its straight for and proven.

There is no magic formula, but there are a few things that will make the process easier.

Part 1
Mental Body-Fat

*"Losing body-fat may be just as much
mental as physical!"*

I
Balance

"You have to constantly juggle your mind and body to lower-body fat!"

Solving the whole body-fat thing can be summed up in one word, *"Balance;"* a much easy word to write than to succeed, I must say.

Balance- *"An equality between the sums total of the two sides."* In fitness and body-fat there are a few more sides of the equation than just two.

Never Ending Challenge

I was not in a very good mood yesterday and I stated the following to one of my clients, *"If you think for one second that you will work really hard, reach a goal and all will be perfect, you are sorely mistaken and will in the end be very disappointed."*

The same attitude must apply to acquiring an ideal body fat level over time. You must take a life long, day to day approach. Balancing anything in life is usually the biggest challenge any of us will every have. Add the balancing of the ideal workout and eating plan to normal life and it can be doubly as challenging.

The Approach

When I first started workout I had ZERO discipline, faith in myself or confidence that I would or could succeed. Fortunately for some reason I just believed this, *"If I could just get through one day, and one day only at a time then I would worry about tomorrow, well, tomorrow."*

The Attitude

Not to jump ahead but I also learned over time that having a balanced workout, eating and life plan all the time was pretty much impossible. When one area of the plan is doing well, you have to shift gears to another area. When that one is under control then either the first one or another totally different area of your life and fitness plan needs to be worked on.

My point is this, the goal to lower your body fat is to achieve as close to a balanced plan of all the important things as one possibly can. However, you need to understand that you will never get it perfect, nor if you think you have it, then it will not take long before an area needs more tweaking. You will always be seeking a balanced approach to fitness. The closer you get to it, and the longer you can achieve it, the lower your body-fat will go and stay.

The Area's

There are three main areas I want to focus on in this e book. Each one does not work with out the other. Like a spoke in a wheel with out one the tire will go flat; so goes your body-fat. The three main areas are: Psychology, Nutrition and Physical Training.

Again, allow me to challenge you to take a long term approach, and an attitude that each day will be a constant balancing act of all three areas.

II
Body vs. Mind

"Lowering body-fat takes more faith at times than fitness!"

While a balanced approach is the key, I never said it would be easy. Maintaining the momentum and synergy of everything may come down to more mental than physical. The challenge with the whole subject of body-fat is we can't see it totally. You can look good, but still have less than desirable body-fat levels. The goal is to keep the EGO in check; easier said than done.

Mirrors and Clothes Don't Lie

Man or woman it doesn't matter the mind and EGO is an internal competitor; for woman its vanity, for men it's about being moncho. You can very easily get off base by focusing too much on looks, or bench press numbers, rather than the levels of fat you have.

I've always tried to express to people that at the end of the day, the mirror and clothes don't lie; meaning those two things probably are more accurate of your over all health than a scale.

Chances are if your clothes are feeling loser then your body-fat is most likely decreasing; not always though.

What you can't see may kill you

Diabetes is one of the fastest growing diseases today. On some level it seems as though you wake up one morning and you have it; that's really not the case. Developing Diabetes is a process that takes time. Poor eating habits, lack of exercise and genetics all contribute to such a disease. Not being able to see the development of diabetes in our bodies makes us not take it so serious or even increase a state of denial.

The chance's of getting diabetes in your body has been there for some time, but it was not visual so it never crossed your mind. One morning you awake and the doctor says, "Yep, you got it." Diabetes is caused by high levels of body-fat by the way.

You take a similar approach to your body-fat levels, if you can't see it then you assume it's not a problem, or worse yet, not even on the radar screen of life.

Body Fat-Thin is NOT In

Thin is NOT in! When I worked for Kathy Smith in Los Angeles, California I managed about fifty employees; ten of them were aerobic instructors.

Out of the ten half weighed an average of 115 pounds. The shocking thing was come to find out through a club testing day most of them were clinically considered obese. What? How can that be? By looking at them you would draw the conclusion that they were in great shape; and to the public eye they were.

Thin is NOT In

The tests discovered that over thirty percent of their total body weight was in the form of fat, medically, making them fit into the obese category; totally shocking to the naked eye. So be very careful not to distort the idea that thinness equals healthiness.

In short for the instructors, to high heart rate over time ate away at muscle tissue, combined with poor eating habits eventually made their ratio of muscle to overall body weight out of balance.

Contrast this with some football players who are big and bulky and the same thing occurs, too much weight and a decrease in muscle can make you obese with out looking like it.

Part 2
Physical Body-Fat

*"Understanding what body-fat is and the
importance of lowering it is half the battle!"*

III
Body-Fat

"Getting muscular or losing weight is one thing, lowering your body-fat is another story!"

What is Body-Fat?

Body fat is a compound comprised of glycerol -- a substance formed in fatty acids -- and fatty acids which is required as a concentrated energy source for our muscles. Fat is a storage substance for the body's extra calories and it fills fat cells (adipose tissue) that help insulate the body. When the body has used up the calories from carbohydrates it begins to depend on the calories from fat.

How can I determine body fat percentage?

There are several ways to find out your body fat percentage. Unfortunately, the more accurate the method, the more of a hassle and/or expensive it tends to be.

DEXA scan – full body X-ray scan of the same type used for bone density. Very accurate.

Hydrostatic Weighing – Weighing under water (completely submerged, with all air blown out of lungs) – Very accurate when done professionally.

Skin-fold calipers ("pinch test") – Simple, but needs to be done by someone who is trained, and you can't do it on yourself. Wide variations in accuracy for people without training.

Bioelectrical Impedance (BIA) – These are scales and hand-held devises that run low-level (and painless) electrical current through you. They can be accurate, although the accuracy varies according to the specific device (do your research) and how it is used.

Best results are obtained first thing in the morning with no alcohol consumed for 2 days prior, and no exercise the night before.

Navy tape measure method - This is a formula based on several body measurements taken with a tape measure. It can be quite accurate (it is used by the military), but it does depend upon your ability to accurately measure. Using centimeters rather than inches is the best, but using inches within ¼ of an inch works. To be sure, measure yourself 3 times and take the average.

What's the difference between Body Fat Percentage and BMI?

BMI (body mass index) is a formula based on height and weight. It was developed because in the general population, it is correlated with body fat. However, there are quite a few groups of people for whom BMI is not as accurate -- short women and muscular people, to name two.

BMI also varies according to some ethnic groups. Also, for people who are interested in changing their body composition and not just their weight, knowing body fat percentage is an improvement over BMI. For example, if you are exercising to build muscle (a good goal), knowing your body fat percentage is a good idea.

Also, when losing weight, you want to preserve as much lean body mass as possible. (Low-carb diets generally produce better results than high carb ones for this purpose.)

If you want to lose or gain weight, you need to be able to measure the state your body is in now and then monitor the changes as you add or subtract calories from your diet. One way to do this is to calculate and monitor your Body Mass Index (BMI).

Since a typical scale only measures your total weight, it helps to have more information to determine if that weight is healthy or unhealthy. A person who is six feet tall and weighs 198 pounds is probably going to have a smaller amount of body fat than a person who is five feet tall and 198 pounds.

The BMI combines your weight and your height into a score that helps you determine if you are underweight, at a healthy weight, overweight, or obese.

BMI is calculated with the following formula:

weight (lb) / [height (in)]^2 x 703 or in

metric:weight (kg) / [height (m)]^2

What Your BMI Means

You can compare your BMI to this table to help you determine whether you're at a healthy weight.

- Underweight = less than 18.5

- Normal weight = 18.5-24.9

- Overweight = 25-29.9

- Obese = 30 or greater

If you are planning to lose or gain weight, you can use your BMI to monitor your progress. It's important to know that your BMI is not the same as your body fat percentage, which is a different number and doesn't correspond to these charts.

People who have a BMI in the overweight or obese ranges may have a higher risk of cardiovascular disease, diabetes, arthritis, and some forms of cancer. However, it's important to see your health care provider, who can take other lifestyle and risk factors into consideration.

The BMI isn't perfect because it's an indirect measurement of fat, and really doesn't differentiate pounds of fat from pounds of muscle and bone. So it doesn't work well for very muscular people or for people who have lost a lot of muscle mass.

For example, an elite athlete with a very small amount of body fat will still have a high BMI, and an elderly person may have a lower BMI because they have less muscle mass. In these cases, a better method of measurement is the body fat percentage.

By the Numbers

If you are a numbers person here are ones to shoot for when trying to lower your body fat.

Age	Under fat	Healthy Range	Overweight	Obese
20-40 yrs	Under 21%	21-33%	33-39%	Over 39
41-60 yrs	Under 23%	23-35%	35-40%	Over 40
61-79 yrs	Under 24%	24-36%	36-42%	Over 42

Men

Age	Under fat	Healthy Range	Overweight	Obese
20-40 yrs	Under 8%	8-19%	19-25%	Over 25
41-60 yrs	Under 11%	11-22%	22-27%	Over 27
61-79 yrs	Under 13%	13-25%	25-30%	Over 30

Above Average Below Grade

Unfortunately most of you are above the average, and in the body-fat category anything above is not good. So what grade will you give yourself?

There are many things that contribute to higher body-fat but in this book we will only concentrate on a few of the things that will give you more bang for the buck. For me there a few major things that I concentrated on daily that helped me keep my body-fat low for years.

IV
Blood Sugar

"Blood Sugar, Food and Training- The Ultimate Goal!"

For the last twenty five years or so I have had one daily goal. I found by achieving this goal each day, my body-fat would stay at a lower level. I understood that if I monitored and regulated my blood sugar levels through good nutritional habits, and a balanced exercise program the rest would kind of fall into place.

What is Blood Sugar?

In short, blood **sugar** concentration or blood glucose level **is** the amount of glucose (**sugar**) present in the blood.

Blood sugar, also known as blood glucose, is the body's fuel that feeds the brain, nervous system, and tissues. A healthy body makes glucose not only from ingested carbohydrates, but also from proteins and fats, and would not be able to function without it. Maintaining a balanced blood glucose level is essential to a body's everyday performance.

Glucose is absorbed directly into the bloodstream from the intestine and results in a rapid increase in the blood glucose level. The pancreas releases insulin, a natural hormone, to prevent blood glucose levels from excessively elevating, and aids in the moving of glucose into the cells. Glucose is then carried to each cell, providing them with the energy needed to carry out its specific function.

Healthy blood glucose levels are considered to be in the 70-120 range. One high or low reading does not always indicate a problem, but the glucose level should be monitored for 10-14 days. There are several different tests that can be administered to determine whether an individual has a problem maintaining a normal glucose level such as: a fasting blood sugar test, an oral glucose test, or a random blood sugar test. Blood glucose levels that remain either too high or too low over time may cause damage to the eyes, kidneys, nerves and blood vessels.

Hypoglycemia

Hypoglycemia is a condition caused by low blood sugar levels in the body, can be extremely debilitating if not controlled properly. Symptoms include shaking, irritability, confusion, strange behavior and even loss of consciousness. These symptoms can be corrected by ingesting a form of a sugar such as a hard candy, a sugar pill, or a sweet drink. Ingesting one or more of these forms of sugar quickly raises the body's blood sugar level and has an almost immediate effect.

Hyperglycemia

Hyperglycemia occurs when the blood glucose levels in the body are higher than normal. Symptoms of this condition include: excessive thirst, frequent urination, tiredness, weakness and lethargy. If the levels become excessively high, a person can become dehydrated and comatose.

A Side Note

Diabetes occurs when the pancreas either produces little or no insulin, or the cells do not respond appropriately to the insulin produced. There are three main types of diabetes: Type 1 , Type 2, and Gestational Diabetes. Type 1 diabetes occurs when the body's immune system attacks insulin producing cells in the pancreas destroying them and causing the pancreas to produce little or no insulin. Type 2 diabetes is the most common and is associated with age, obesity, and genetics.

Gestational diabetes develops only during pregnancy, but means an increase in the chance of the woman developing Type 2 diabetes in the future. All types of diabetes are serious and need to be monitored regularly.

Insulin Resistance

What is insulin resistance?

Insulin resistance is a condition in which the body produces insulin but does not use it properly. Insulin, a hormone made by the pancreas, helps the body use glucose for energy. Glucose is a form of sugar that is the body's main source of energy.

The body's digestive system breaks food down into glucose, which then travels in the bloodstream to cells throughout the body. Glucose in the blood is called blood glucose, also known as blood sugar. As the blood glucose level rises after a meal, the pancreas releases insulin to help cells take in and use the glucose.

When people are insulin resistant, their muscle, fat, and liver cells do not respond properly to insulin. As a result, their bodies need more insulin to help glucose enter cells. The pancreas tries to keep up with this increased demand for insulin by producing more. Eventually, the pancreas fails to keep up with the body's need for insulin.

Excess glucose builds up in the bloodstream, setting the stage for diabetes. Many people with insulin resistance have high levels of both glucose and insulin circulating in their blood at the same time.

Insulin resistance increases the chance of developing type 2 diabetes and heart disease. Learning about insulin resistance is the first step toward making lifestyle changes that can help prevent diabetes and other health problems.

What causes insulin resistance?

Scientists have identified specific genes that make people more likely to develop insulin resistance and diabetes. Excess weight and lack of physical activity also contribute to insulin resistance.

Many people with insulin resistance and high blood glucose have other conditions that increase the risk of developing type 2 diabetes and damage to the heart and blood vessels, also called cardiovascular disease.

These conditions include having excess weight around the waist, high blood pressure, and abnormal levels of cholesterol and triglycerides in the blood. Having several of these problems is called metabolic syndrome or insulin resistance syndrome, formerly called syndrome X.

Roller (coaster)

A good indicator (or one for me) that my blood sugar levels were off during the day was my tiredness around mid morning and afternoon.

If you look at roller coasters you will basically find two kinds; hilly ones and those that just go straight up and down. Or maybe we could visualize a one hump camel or a two humped one. Either way, the goals is to not have too many humps (ups and downs) in your blood sugar levels through out the day.

Two Humped Camels

When your blood sugar levels, or energy levels go up and down like a two humped camel you DO NOT burn body-fat. Chances are you will probably do the opposite of what you should do. (See the nutritional chapter)

The Five Hour Energy Craze

Each year American's consume about eight hundred million dollars of the product called, "Five Hour Energy Drink."

Why, because, most people are tired either mid morning or mid afternoon? The drink apparently revives you long enough (five hours) to get through the rest of your day. All it is, is caffeine and mineral water. The company is basically making boat loads of money off of people's LAZINESS.

I really believe that people's biggest problem of obesity and high body-fat levels is due to poor regulation of their blood sugars caused by lack of exercise and poor eating habits.

Blood Sugar Regulation

Blood sugar levels are regulated by negative feedback in order to keep the body in homeostasis.

The levels of glucose in the blood are monitored by the cells in the pancreas's Islets of Langerhans.

If the blood glucose level falls to dangerous levels (as in very heavy exercise or lack of food for extended periods), the Alpha cells of the pancreas release glucagon, a hormone whose effects on liver cells act to increase blood glucose levels.

They convert glycogen into glucose (this process is called glycogenolysis). The glucose is released into the bloodstream, increasing blood sugar levels.

While far as I know I am not diabetic or even pre-diabetic, however for me the whole ball of wax came down to, *"HOW do I control and regulate my blood sugar levels every single day?"* It came down to two categories; eating and exercising smart.

Here are a few ways I regulated by blood sugar levels:

- Eat often
- Never skip breakfast
- Don't eat past 8 at night
- No white flour at noon or evening meals
- Protein snacks between meals
- Workout in the morning

Part 3
Consumable Body-Fat

"Balance the diet and solve your body-fat issue, half way!"

V
Binging- Portion Control

"Control the roller coaster and cure the body-fat!"

Call it any thing you want, but eating to much food in too little time in my mind is binging; and binging cause blood sugar problems which in the long run raises body-fat levels.

If you really want to know how much you are eating, just calculate all the calories you consume in a day, or in each meal at the very least. I would be willing to bet you would be surprised and even shocked at the amount of calories consumed or inhaled.

You always hear about snacking and eating smaller meals through out the day, why? By nature we eat more when we eat less often.

One feeds on the other

We talked about blood sugar levels and the important of keeping them even through out the day, but it also must be noted how low blood sugar levels promote bigger portion sizes, in turn larger portion sizes spike blood sugar levels and then they crash. Each one feeds on the other building up so much momentum that in some cases if you don't exercise you run the risk of becoming pre-diabetic or worse full blown diabetes.

VI
Before Noon
"Early bird gets the energy"

If I have any secrets to keeping my body fat lower than most here's one of them; I front load my carbohydrates daily.

Carbohydrate FRONT Loading

What the heck do you mean Front loading your carbohydrates?

Let's look at the habits of most people. One reason so many people have gotten fatter over the years is because of convenience, laziness and lack of planning their foods. What food group is the easiest to get and fix? Yes, carbohydrates. And when do people eat the majority of those carbohydrates, at night, right? What do carbohydrates supply to the body? Yes, energy. When do we need the most energy, at night or in the morning? So, what's wrong with this picture then?

Eating good food can still make you fat

In the early nineties a study came out on how good pasta was for you, so what did people do? They ate more pasta.

American's are almost twenty percent fatter today than back then. How can that be, pasta was suppose to be good for you? It is, however, consumed at night followed by a night on your back, converts into glucose and over time, fat.

Front Loading

You hear of carbohydrate loading in sports so I guess you could say that I carbohydrates loaded to keep my body-fat low. Well a better and more accurate way of saying it is, I FRONT loaded my carbohydrate intake. In other words, if I want to keep my body-fat lower I will eat the majority of my carbohydrates, more importantly the complex carbs prior to the two o'clock hour.

Part 4
Training to Lower Body-Fat

"Physical exercise is like a tool of a sculpture, if used just enough, art is created!"

VII
Beliefs from the Core

"Having a little faith may be the most important action to lower body-fat!"

The core muscle groups may be the most functional and important muscle groups in your body. They also may be the most neglected out of them all as well.

Your Belief System

One thing I learned early on in my body building career was that you have to have a strong belief in working out your core muscles. It's very easy to make any excuse NOT to exercise the core muscles.

The other thing is, they HURT. Doing core muscle group exercises are painful, so you have to believe in what you are doing at the time, a little faith goes along ways.

Faith

Having faith in something you can't see is challenging to say the least. Just looking at your body in the mirror is no accurate way of measuring body-fat. You can't even muster a good guess by a visual.

VIII
Blood Work

In the beginning chapter of this book we discussed the importance of being balanced. When it comes to physical training to lower your body-fat it's a dicey path. It really is a balancing act of good food, sleep, a stress free attitude, cardiovascular and strength training. The goal is to rid the body of fat while at the same time continue to develop lean muscle tissue.

Blood Flow- Cardiovascular Training

Just walking, biking, crossfit or step class does not cut it when it comes to losing weight and body-fat. I can not remember the last I went into a gym and saw a member check their heart rate zone.

Target Heart Rate Zone

There is no way you will get to your ideal body-fat weight unless you hit your target heart rate zone every time you perform cardiovascular training; don't go over or under, you have to hit the target.

If you go over you burn valuable muscle, under and weight stays on. Memorize this formula;

220-age x 60-85% = Target Heart Rate (THR)

Cardiovascular Training Protocol

Like I said, I never see people take their heart rates, machine or by hand. So here is the protocol you should follow to lower the fat levels efficiently:

1. First and fore most calculate your heart rate numbers. You only have to do this once and memorize the zone and divide by six.
2. No matter what cardiovascular piece of equipment you use by the seven minute mark of your workout you should and must be in your zone. Most people are not in there until twelve to fifteen minutes in.
3. Maintain this zone for a minimum of twenty minutes and a maximum of forty minutes.

4.   Don't just get off of the equipment at the end, slow the pace down gradually; this is the cool-down period. Cardiac arrest may occur if you don't cool down properly.

Cannibalism

Cannibals eat their own. If you exercise with your heart rate to high your muscles eat their own.

The average weight of my aerobic instructors in LA was around 115 pounds. After a surprise body-fat test, over half were clinically obese. How is that possible? Cannibalism!

Day after day they failed to monitor their heart rates, thus they were too high. Day after day their bodies were not being fueled properly for their training regiment. With the combination of the two, their body's recuperation process could not keep up with the demand they had been putting on themselves.

Over time, precious muscle tissue was being eaten away like hungry, desperate pack man. Eventually, the percentage of body-fat to their over all weight was close or over thirty percent, clinically obese numbers. Ouch!

More is not better either!

Don't make the mistake of trying to put logic with exercise, your dealing with a human body that in the end will not be able to totally manipulate. Those aerobic instructors for some reason thought that the more they did, the higher they kept their heart rates the less they would weight and lower the body-fat. Unfortunately, all that did was hurt their health not help it.

Cycle Intensity Levels

Adaptation is a word you will hear me say frequently. I truly believe the body is smart and has a good memory. This will take some pre-planning on your part, however, maybe one of the smartest and most effective techniques I have used in keeping my body-fat low over the years.

In other words, never do the same identical cardiovascular workout three times in a row. This can be accomplished by changing length of workouts, elevations or intensity levels, time during the day or even locations.

IX
Body Work

Cardiovascular is aerobic and weight training is anaerobic, we all know this, however, there is one little thing I have discovered over the years when it comes to weight training and body-fat.

We are all taught as well as you have learned in this book that a combination of food, cardiovascular and now weight training aids in lowering body-fat. Now let's dissect this theory a little bit more in detail as it pertains to weight training and body-fat.

Flipping the Switch

I truly believe that you can keep your body-fat lower over time more so than even most people imagine as it pertains to weights. Not so much the exercises, but the technique in which you go through the workouts. Over the years I learned to flip a switch right before I walked into the gym.

Time Lines

The first thing I did was, decide to put a time limit to my weight training workouts.
Whether I was done with my body-parts or not I would walk out of the gym. Walking out once or twice cured me of messing around.

The Art of Flow

I have been complimented time and time again for how artful my workouts look. From afar there seems to be a sense of methodical flow from rep to set, exercise to machine; an effortless motion. Like I mentioned, flipping the mental switch and times lines cut my time down between sets and exercises and in the long run by doing this my body-fat stayed lower.

Call it, flow, intensity, focus what ever you want to, all I know is, body-fat stayed off, I had more fun and received more results in a shorter period of time.

X
Bonus

Variety

I am convinced that our bodies get bored with what we do physically, adapt and plateau in getting results. Mentally we get stale and that translates into physical stagnation. Then what do you do? You quit.

Pre Planning

Putting variety into your workouts and eating habits takes a little thinking ahead; this is why most don't do it, its too much work. However, pre-planning your workouts and eating accomplishes two things, takes a lot of wasted energy and time out of your life and builds confidence, which in turn creates momentum.

Workout Variety

Our bodies start getting use to repetitive actions with in our workouts around six to eight weeks into a workout plan.

I really can not explain it, but the body assumes you are going to do the same exercise, weight and order of those exercises after a certain time. When this happens the body plateaus and in some cases the body fat goes up, because the heart rate stays at a lower rate through out the workout.

Food Variety

Maybe it's the typical number of calories, I'm not sure but just as with a typical workout for you the body gets use to the same old foods you eat as well. If you have oatmeal and wheat toast every morning for breakfast even though the food types are good for you the calorie amount stays the same. Over time the body gets use to that amount of calories and again, the metabolism slows down.

Conclusion

For overall health stand point, there is nothing more valuable than keeping your body-fat in check. If you are concerned about appearance, a body never looks better than lean and mean. Achieving such a goal is not as hard as *keeping* ones body-fat lower; it really does take a *balanced* approach.

In my opinion, it's easy to put on muscle or lose weight, but it's much more difficult to do both at the same time; its quality not quantity. Quality muscle and low body mass takes a juggling act on a consistent basis and in the end it maybe more of a *mind* game than anything.

In order to over come something you have to understand what it is and why its there. Body-fat is not Body Mass. Body-fat is not necessarily pounds read on a scale either.

Remember to keep the first things first, and always focus on *blood sugar*. If you regulate your blood sugar the body-fat has to stay low. I realize life is hectic these days, however some way some how you have to *pre plan*, set goals and be proactive verses reactive. If you don't, you will constantly eat more than you should, throwing your metabolism into a free fall.

Body-fat tends to come off easier when the metabolism stays constant through out the day not the evening so watch those high energy foods late at night. You have to realize that it's not all about exercise, it's about food too. But when you do exercise more is NOT better. Be smart, efficient and precise. Monitor your efforts, structure with variety works best for me. You do all this one day you will awake and guess what, the switch is flipped and the body-fat has gone.

Its not rocket science, but it will take work. And I know you've heard this a lot, but seriously, if I've done this you can too; one goal, one day, one meal, one workout, one percent body-fat at a time.

Good Luck!

Greg Ryan

Website: www.resolutions.bz
Email: greg@resolutions.bz

I have a wealth of FREE information on weight loss, fitness, nutrition and bodybuilding.

Website: www.resolutions.bz
Email: greg@resolutions.bz

FREE Fitness Advice

Blogs:

www.resolutionsblog.com

www.reso-care.com

www.gregryanfitness.com

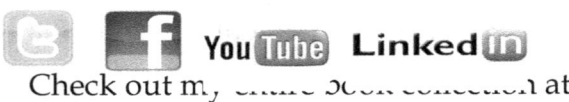

Check out m, ... Jook ....1 at

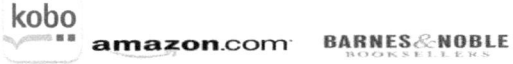